PULMONAI
TREATMEN

The Ultimate Remedy Guide On Understanding The Disease, Managing Your Symptoms And Navigating Treatment

DR. JERRY SAMSON

Table of Contents

CHAPTER ONE

Pulmonary Embolism

Sudden shortness of breath, pain in and around the chest, and coughing are all signs of a pulmonary embolism and should be taken seriously. A pulmonary embolism is a serious but extremely manageable ailment that is caused by a blood clot and should be treated as soon as possible.

A pulmonary embolism is a blockage in one of the pulmonary arteries in your lungs that causes blood to pool in the lungs. In the majority of cases, pulmonary embolism is caused by blood clots that move to the lungs from deep veins in the legs or, in rare situations, from veins in other parts of the body, according to the American Heart Association (deep vein thrombosis).

Pulmonary embolism is a potentially life-threatening condition because the clots prevent blood from flowing to the lungs. Early treatment, on the other hand, significantly reduces the risk of mortality. Taking precautions to avoid blood clots in your legs will assist to protect you from a pulmonary embolism in the future.

What is a pulmonary embolism, and how does it happen?

An embolism (blood clot in the lung) is a blood clot in the lung that develops when a blood clot in another region of the body (usually the leg or arm) travels through the bloodstream and becomes stuck in the blood vessels of the lung (pulmonary embolism). This reduces blood flow to the lungs, lowers oxygen levels in the lungs, and raises blood pressure in the pulmonary arteries, all of which have negative consequences.

A thrombus is a blood clot that forms in a vein and remains there for an extended period of time. It is referred to as an embolus if the blood clot breaks away from the wall of the vein and moves to another portion of your body.

If PEs are not treated promptly, they can result in heart or lung damage, as well as death in some cases.

What types of people are at risk of acquiring a blood clot?

A blood clot is more likely to form in people who have been inactive or immobile for an extended length of time, such as those who have been on bed rest or have had surgery.

A personal or family history of blood clotting disorders, such as deep vein thrombosis (DVT) or pulmonary embolism (PE), is a risk factor (PE).

• Have a family history of cancer or are currently undergoing chemotherapy

• Sit for extended periods of time.

People who are at risk for getting a pulmonary embolism include those who: • are inactive for extended periods of time while traveling by car, rail, or airline; and

• Have a family history of heart failure or a stroke, or both.

• Have a body mass index of 30 or higher.

• Have recently had trauma or injury to a vein, which could have occurred as a result of a recent operation, fracture, or varicose veins.

- Are pregnant or have recently given birth within the last six weeks.

Have you recently started using birth control tablets (oral contraceptives) or hormone replacement therapy?

Installation of central venous catheters through an arm or leg. You should speak with your health-care provider if you have any of these risk factors and have previously experienced a blood clot so that efforts can be taken to minimize your unique risk.

What is the severity of a pulmonary embolism?

When appropriately detected and treated, a pulmonary embolism has a low chance of becoming life-threatening. Left untreated, on the other hand, it can become life-threatening, resulting in additional medical concerns, even death. In addition to causing heart damage, a pulmonary embolism can be life-threatening depending on the size of the blood clot.

CHAPTER TWO

Symptoms

Because the amount of lung tissue affected by a pulmonary embolism, the size of the clots, and whether or not you have an underlying lung or heart condition all influence the severity of the symptoms.

• Shortness of breath is one of the most common indications and symptoms. If you have this symptom, it will usually appear unexpectedly and will always worsen with exertion.

• Aches and pains in the chest. Perhaps you're experiencing symptoms of a heart attack. In many cases, the pain is intense and felt when you take a deep breath, and it prevents you from taking another deep breath. Coughing, bending, and stooping can all cause it to be felt.

• Cough. Coughing may result in the production of bloody or blood-streaked sputum.

Other indications and symptoms that can arise as a result of a pulmonary embolism are as follows:

Deep vein thrombosis (DVT) symptoms include: rapid or irregular heartbeat; lightheadedness or dizziness; excessive sweating; fever; leg discomfort or swelling, or both, generally in the calves; clammy or discolored skin (cyanosis)

When should you visit the doctor?

Pulmonary embolism is a serious medical condition that can be fatal. If you feel unexplained shortness of breath, chest pain, or a cough that produces bloody sputum, seek medical attention right once.

Causes

It is possible to suffer from an embolism of the lung if you have an accumulation of material, most commonly a blood clot, lodged in an artery in your lung. Deep vein thrombosis is a disorder in which blood clots form in the deep veins of your legs, which is the most prevalent source of these blood clots (DVT).

In many cases, pulmonary embolism is caused by a collection of blood clots. The regions of the lungs serviced by each clogged artery are deprived of blood and may perish as a result of the blockage. A pulmonary infarction is the medical term for this. It becomes more difficult for your lungs to give oxygen to the rest of your body as a result of this condition.

There are also instances in which blockages in the blood vessels are produced by items other than blood clots. These include: • Fat from the marrow of a shattered long bone • A tumor or a tumor fragment • Air bubbles

CHAPTER THREE

Factors that increase risk

Despite the fact that anyone can develop blood clots and a resulting pulmonary embolism, there are some factors that can enhance your risk.

Medical conditions and therapies are discussed.

In the past, you or a member of your family may have suffered from deep vein thrombosis (DVT) or pulmonary embolism, which increases your risk.

In addition, certain medical disorders and therapies, such as the following, put you at risk:

• Coronary artery disease. Clot development is increased in the presence of cardiovascular illness, specifically heart failure.

• Cancer. Brain, ovarian, pancreatic, colon, stomach, lung and kidney cancers are among the tumors that can raise the risk of blood clots. Chemotherapy can also increase the risk of blood clots in patients with cancer that has spread. Women who have a personal or family history of breast cancer and are taking tamoxifen or raloxifene are at an increased risk of developing blood clots as well.

• Surgery. Surgery is one of the most common causes of blood clots that create problems. It is for this reason that anticoagulant medicine may be administered before and after major surgery, such as joint replacement.

• Disorders that have an impact on coagulation. A number of hereditary illnesses have an effect on the blood, making it more susceptible to clot formation. Other medical conditions, such as kidney illness, can raise your chance of developing blood clots as well.

• Coronavirus disease in the year 2019 (COVID-19). People who suffer from severe COVID-19 symptoms are at an elevated risk of developing a pulmonary embolism.

Immobility for an extended period of time

Inactivity, such as bed rest, increases the likelihood of blood clots forming in the blood vessels. Being confined to your bed for an extended amount of time following surgery, a heart attack, a limb fracture, a traumatic injury, or any significant sickness increases your risk of developing blood clots in your lungs. When the lower limbs are kept horizontal for extended periods of time, the flow of venous blood slows, causing blood to pool in the legs and, in certain cases, blood clots to form.

• Extensive travel. Sitting in a confined space for long periods of time on a plane or in a car causes blood flow in the legs to slow, which leads to the formation of clots.

Other potential dangers
• Smoking. Tobacco use, for reasons that are not fully

understood, predisposes some persons to the formation of blood clots, especially when paired with other risk factors.

• Having a large waist circumference. Excess weight raises the chance of blood clots, especially in persons who already have other risk factors for the condition.

• Hormone replacement therapy. It is possible that the estrogen found in birth control pills and hormone replacement treatment will raise the levels of clotting factors in your blood, especially if you smoke or are overweight.

• Pregnancy. The pressure of the baby resting on veins in the pelvis might cause blood flow from the legs to be delayed. When blood slows or pools, it increases the likelihood of clot formation.

CHAPTER FOUR

Complications

Pulmonary embolism is a serious medical condition that can be fatal. Undiagnosed and untreated pulmonary embolisms result in the death of around one-third of those who suffer from them. When the condition is diagnosed and treated as soon as possible, however, the number of cases drops significantly.

An embolism in the lungs can also result in pulmonary hypertension, which is a condition in which the blood pressure in your lungs and on the right side of your heart is abnormally elevated. In the presence of obstructions in the arteries that provide blood to the lungs, your heart has to work harder to push blood through the vessels, raising your blood pressure and ultimately weakening your heart.

Small emboli occur often in rare cases and grow in size over time, leading in chronic pulmonary hypertension, also known as chronic thromboembolic pulmonary hypertension, in the affected lungs.

Prevention

Preventing blood clots in the deep veins of your legs (deep vein thrombosis) will assist to reduce the risk of pulmonary embolism and other complications. As a result, most hospitals are vigorous in their efforts to prevent blood clots, employing procedures such as: • Blood thinners (anticoagulants). These medications are frequently prescribed to patients who are at risk of blood clots before and after an operation, as well as to those who are admitted to the hospital with medical problems such as heart attack, stroke, or cancer-related complications.

• Compression stockings are a type of compression stocking. With continuous pressure applied to your legs, compression stockings aid in the efficient flow of blood through your veins and leg muscles. They provide a safe, easy, and low-cost method of preventing blood from stagnating during and after common surgical procedures.

• Elevation of the legs. Elevating your legs whenever possible, especially during the night, can be extremely beneficial. Blocks or books can be used to raise the bottom of your bed by 4 to 6 inches (10 to 15 cm).

• Participation in physical activities. Moving around as soon as possible after surgery can assist to reduce the risk of pulmonary embolism and speed up the recovery process overall. This is one of the primary reasons your nurse may encourage you to get up and move even on the day of your operation, despite the fact that you are experiencing pain at the site of your surgical incision.

• Pneumatic compression is a type of compression. To massage and squeeze the veins in your legs and promote blood flow, this treatment uses thigh-high or calf-high cuffs that automatically inflate with air and deflate every few minutes.

Precautions should be taken when traveling.

The chance of getting blood clots when traveling is modest, but it increases as the length of time spent traveling grows. In the event that you have risk factors for blood clots and are concerned about traveling, you should consult your doctor.

In order to assist prevent blood clots when traveling, your doctor may recommend the following measures:

• Make sure to drink plenty of fluids. When it comes to reducing dehydration, which can lead to the development of blood clots, water is the greatest liquid to drink. Avoid consuming alcohol, which increases the risk of fluid loss.

• Take a break from sitting for a while. Every hour or so, take a walk around the airplane cabin to clear your head. Whenever you're driving, take a few minutes to get out of the car and walk around it a couple of times. Do a few deep knee bends to warm up.

• Move about in your seat. Every 15 to 30 minutes, flex your ankles to keep them flexible.

• Support stockings should be worn. In order to improve circulation and fluid mobility in your legs, your doctor may prescribe these medications. A variety of fashionable colors and textures are available in compression stockings. There are even gadgets, referred to as stocking butlers, that assist you in putting on your stockings.

CHAPTER FIVE

What are the symptoms of a pulmonary embolism?

Pulmonary embolism is frequently discovered by the use of the following procedures:

• A computed tomography (CT) scan is performed.

• A pulmonary scan.

• Laboratory tests such as blood tests (including the D-dimer test).

• A pulmonary angiography is performed.

In patients who are unable to have an X-ray due to dye allergies or who are too unwell to leave their hospital room, ultrasound of the leg can aid in the detection of blood clots in the legs.

Medical imaging procedures such as magnetic resonance imaging (MRI) of the legs or lungs.

What is the treatment for pulmonary embolism?

It is customary for patients with pulmonary emboli to get treatment in a hospital setting where their condition may be regularly monitored.

The length of your therapy and hospital stay will be determined by the severity of the blood clot that you have.

Based on your medical condition, treatment options may include anticoagulant (blood-thinning) medications, thrombolytic therapy, compression stockings, and occasionally surgery or interventional procedures to improve blood flow and reduce the risk of future blood clots. Anticoagulant (blood-thinning) medications are used to reduce the risk of blood clots.

Anticoagulant medicines are prescribed.

The majority of the time, anti-coagulant drugs are used to treat the condition (also called blood thinners). Anticoagulants work by decreasing the blood's ability to clot and so preventing further blood clot formation.

Warfarin (Coumadin®), heparin, low-molecular-weight heparin (such as Lovenox® or Dalteparin®), and fondaparinux (Arixtra®) are examples of anticoagulant drugs.

• Warfarin is available in tablet form and is administered orally (by mouth).

In hospitals, heparin is administered either through an intravenous (IV) line, which delivers medication directly into the vein, or through subcutaneous (under the skin) injections, which transport medication directly into the bloodstream.

Injections of low molecular-weight heparin are given just beneath or under the skin (subcutaneously). It is given once or twice a day and can be taken at the convenience of the patient's home.

A new medicine, fondaparinux (Arixtra), is administered once a day through a subcutaneous injection into the muscle.

You and your family will receive more advice on how to properly administer the anticoagulant medication that has been prescribed. It is critical, as with any drug, that you understand how and when to take your anticoagulant, as well as that you adhere to your doctor's recommendations.

This is determined by your diagnosis, which determines the sort of medication provided, the length of time you must take it, and the type of follow-up monitoring you will require. It is essential that you attend all scheduled follow-up meetings with your doctor and the laboratory so that your reaction to the drug can be closely monitored and evaluated.

Following treatment with anticoagulants, you will have frequent blood tests, such as the ones listed below.

Tests for prothrombin time (PT or protime) and International Normalized Ratio (INR) include the following: This measurement will assist your health-care professional in ascertaining the rate at which your blood is clotting and whether your medication dosage needs to be adjusted. If you are taking Coumadin, this test will be used to keep track of your progress.

APT (activated partial thromboplastin time) is a measurement of the time it takes for blood to clot to form clots. If you are taking heparin, you will need to have this test done to keep track of your health.

This assay determines the presence of low molecular-weight heparin in the bloodstream (also known as anti-Xa or heparin).

Unless you are overweight, have renal disease, or are pregnant, it is typically not required to have this test performed on you.

CHAPTER SIX

What other therapy alternatives are available?

Compression stockings are a type of compression stocking.

Using compression stockings (support hose) to improve blood flow in the legs is recommended by your doctor and should be done as directed. The stockings are normally knee-high in length and are designed to compress your legs in order to prevent blood from accumulating in them.

Consult your doctor about how to use your compression stockings, how long to wear them, and how to care for them properly. It is critical to wash compression stockings according to the manufacturer's instructions to avoid harming them.

Procedures

If a pulmonary embolism is life-threatening, or if other therapies are ineffective, your doctor may propose one of the following options: surgery.

It is possible to have the embolus removed through surgery. It is also possible to have a filter installed within the largest vein in the body (the vena cava filter) so that blood clots can be captured before they reach the heart and lungs.

Thrombolytic therapy is a type of medication that helps to dissolve blood clots.

Tissue plasminogen activator (TPA) and other thrombolytic drugs (sometimes known as "clot busters") are used to dissolve the blood clot. It is always recommended that thrombolytics be administered in a hospital setting where the patient can be thoroughly monitored. These medications are only used in specific conditions, such as when a patient's blood pressure is low or when the patient's health is unstable as a result of a pulmonary embolism, and are not recommended for routine usage.

What can I do to avoid a pulmonary embolism?

• Engage in regular physical activity. You should move your arms, legs, and feet for a few minutes every hour if you are confined to bed due to bed rest, rehabilitation from surgery, or extended travel. If you know you will be sitting or standing for extended periods of time, consider wearing compression stockings to help blood flow.

Drink lots of fluids, such as water and juice, but stay away from excessive amounts of alcohol and caffeine.

Even if you are required to remain motionless for extended periods of time, take a few minutes every hour to move around: move your feet and legs, bend your knees, and stand on your tip-toes.

• Do not use tobacco products.

• Avoid crossing your legs at all costs.

• Avoid wearing apparel that is too tight.

• If you are overweight, you should lose weight.

• Elevate your feet for 30 minutes twice a day for better circulation.

If you or any of your family members have had a blood clot, talk to your doctor about ways to lower your risk factors for the condition.

You're getting ready for your appointment

Pulmonary embolism is frequently diagnosed and treated at hospitals, emergency rooms, and urgent care clinics in the earliest stages. If you suspect you may be suffering from a pulmonary embolism, seek medical assistance as soon as possible.

What you can do to help

You might want to make a list that includes the following items:

• In-depth explanations of your signs and symptoms

• Specifics on any recent trips that included long car or plane rides; • A list of all medications you're taking, including vitamins, herbal supplements, and any other supplements, as well as the dosages; • Information on your past medical problems, particularly any recent surgeries or illnesses that kept you bedridden for several days; • Information on any recent journeys that involved long car or plane rides;

• Information about the medical conditions of one's parents or siblings

You may have some questions for the doctor.

Exactly what to expect from your physician

The area around the swollen, sensitive, red, and warm area on your legs will most likely be examined by your doctor during the physical exam to determine whether you have a deep vein clot. In addition, he or she will listen to your heart and lungs and take your blood pressure, and he or she will almost certainly request one or more tests.

What is the course of treatment after a pulmonary embolism?

Make sure you and your doctor have a clear understanding of your post-operative care. Comply with your doctor's instructions to lower your risk of experiencing another pulmonary embolism.

Make sure to attend all scheduled appointments with your doctor and with the laboratory so that your response to prescribed treatments can be tracked.

THE END

Printed in Great Britain
by Amazon